Clean Eating Diet

A 10 Day Diet Plan To Eat Clean, Lose Weight And Supercharge Your Body

By Susan T. Williams

Table of Contents

Introduction

Thank you for downloading 'Clean Eating Diet — A 10 Day Diet Plan To Lose Weight And Supercharge Your Body'

Oftentimes, our bodies deserve a fresh start because over the years we've punished them with bad food and unhealthy habits. We've forgotten how important it is to have a fully functioning body, and we've ignored the health risks that come with eating the wrong foods. Today, I want to talk to you about the Clean Eating Diet, a lifestyle choice that I fully believe will help you to transform your life forever. It's so good to share something with you that means so much to me because after years of not paying any attention to my body, I finally took charge and made a change. Now, I'm healthier and happier than ever before and all because of one simple change in my life — I started eating clean.

More and more, the diet of modern man has unfortunately become very unhealthy, to the point of being dangerous. Even when people think they are being healthy they are often mistaken because clever marketing strategies have changed the way we see certain foods. Over the years, the way we eat has completely changed, and we've all fallen victim to the effects. From obesity to diabetes, high blood pressure to sleep apnea, the list of diseases afflicting the modern man has become far too long, and all of them can be traced back to the foods we are eating.

The problem is that we don't know what goes into most of the food we are eating, and we don't see all the extra sodium, cholesterol, fats and sugar that have gone into making it taste so good. Over time, our bodies have gotten accustomed to eating this way, and in the United States, we've quickly become a nation that's mostly overweight.

Something needs to be done now so that we can regain our health and wellbeing. It's time we started appreciating our bodies more by giving it the nourishment and attention it needs. So how we do we do this?

The basic principle behind clean eating is simple — it's all about going back to our roots. When we look back at how man used to eat, it's easy to see how much things have changed. The ancient man's diet consisted of entirely unprocessed, raw and organic foods that were from the earth instead of from a factory. When food was cooked, it didn't go through any harsh cooking methods and retained its core nutrients. Now, when we cook, the final product is often very different from the natural state of the food. We've gotten so hooked on preservatives and added sugar that we don't know how to eat without them.

When you look at weight statistics over the years, you will clearly see that people starting becoming more and more overweight around the time that processed foods started becoming popular. Before that, obesity was uncommon.

The clean eating diet, which we'll go through in more detail later, is very different from any other diet. For one, it's not a 'fad' but rather a way of eating and living, and the ten day diet plan is simply a way to cleanse your body and introduce you to a new way of thinking about food. It gives you the chance to take a closer look at the foods that you are eating and gives you a better insight to how these foods make you feel.

The rule is that if a food contains chemicals or has undergone any type of processing method, it is best to avoid that food. Also, you have to avoid foods that contain large amounts of sodium and sugar, unless they are naturally present. This change alone will produce a drastic amount of weight loss and a change in the way you look and feel.

Eating clean has become increasingly popular, and celebrities such as Katy Perry and Gwyneth Paltrow now swear by it. Everyone who tries it says the same thing: they never realized how bad they felt before until they started eating clean and they finally knew what it was like to both look and feel good. All of this goes to show just how accustomed we have become to feeling poorly without even realizing it.

The clean eating diet is a war against the production of modern food and a revolution towards a healthier society.

We're going to take you through some easy to follow guidelines and techniques so that you too can transform your life. All we want from you is ten days. In those ten days you'll lose weight, have more energy and you'll finish off looking at food in a whole new and exciting way.

So let's supercharge your body the clean eating way.

CHAPTER 1

The What and the Why

Clean eating involves avoiding processed foods. However, what counts as processed food? How can you tell if a food is processed or not, and therefore unsuitable? What are the elements of processed foods, and why are they bad for you?

Let's start off by taking a closer look at the definition of processed foods. When you are trying to decide whether or not something is processed you just have to ask yourself three basic questions:

Does this food contain any additives?

A food additive is a chemical that has been added to the food in order to change its flavor/appearance or to lengthen the time it can sit on a store shelf. There are many different types of food additives (and the list continues to grow daily), but here are some of the most common ones to look out for when you are doing your grocery shopping:

Artificial sweeteners: Some artificial sweeteners are FDA-regulated, but those generally recognized as safe are not. Some of the artificial sweeteners you should avoid are saccharin, aspartame, high fructose corn syrup, acesulfame potassium, sucralose, agave nectar, bleached starch and tert butlhydroquinone. Many of these sweeteners are linked to cancer, obesity and heart problems.

Artificial food coloring: These are chemical dyes which are used to color food and drinks to make them more pleasing to the eye. While they might make our food look good, there has also been a great deal of research dedicated to what effect they may be having on our bodies. Experts are becoming increasingly aware of the problems that some of these dyes may cause, including increasing the risk of certain cancers and promoting asthma and hyperactivity in children. Most food coloring is derived from petroleum, the same substance we use to power our cars. Here are some artificial food dyes to avoid: red #40, blue #1, blue #2, green #3, orange B, yellow #5 & #6 and red #2 and #3.

Aspartame: This is an artificial sweetener which many people use instead of sugar in their tea and coffee. This is also a common additive in diet soft drinks. It has been said to cause many mental issues such as headaches and seizures.

Azodicarbonamide: Also known as E927 , this is a chemical substance that is used as an agent in certain flours and doughs. According to the FDA, it has been shown to increase the incidence of tumors when fed to female mice.

BHA/BHT: Extending the shelf life of many foods, this fat preservative has been linked to cancer.

Brominated vegetable oil: This particular ingredient, which helps to keep the flavor in oils, does not have to be included on ingredient labels. This is somewhat frightening because it is can cause organ damage if taken in excess.

Butane: This is a very common artificial compound which is used, for example, in chicken nuggets so that they continue to taste fresh, even when they are not. It has also been linked to cancer in animal tests.

Camauba wax: This substance is used in chewing gums and has been linked to cancer and tumors.

Carrageenan: This substance is used in many foods to help with the thickening and stabilization process. It has also been linked to the formation of ulcers and cancer.

Disodium guanylate & disodium inosinate: Both contain MSG. MSG has been linked to headaches, nerve damage, coronary heart disease and seizures.

Enriched flour: This is a very popular refined starch that is used in many foods. Eating products containing enriched white flour causes your body to go through a sugar high/ blood sugar crash cycle. Flour is stripped of its vital nutrients in the manufacturing process and then fortified ingredients that are hard for your body to break down, such as metallic iron, are added back in. It is best to get the nutrients your body needs in their natural state by eating whole grains like rye flour, brown rice flour, millet flour or almond meal.

Estrogen: This hormone is found in all non-organic dairy products. In the modern world of dairy farming, cows are often milked for 300 days a year, much of it while they are pregnant, resulting in much higher levels of estrogen in their milk. In the traditional dairy farms of Mongolia, cows are milked for approximately 5 months a year, resulting in lower estrogen levels. This high rate of estrogen found in most dairy products has been linked to higher rates of cancer in countries where dairy is widely consumed.

MSG: The compound monosodium glutamate is used to enhance the flavor of certain foods. MSG is added to all your potato chips and snack foods to make them palate pleasers. MSG is known for its addictive properties. Its presence in food makes you want to keep going back for more. It has been said that if MSG was added to cardboard, people would want to consume it. MSG stimulates the pancreas to produce more insulin, and because this causes your blood sugar to drop, it means that after eating MSG-laden food, you are hungry within the next hour.

Olestra: This is a substance that is often used to replace natural fats. It is commonly found in snack foods. However, because it is not absorbed properly by the body, it can cause digestive and heart problems.

Parabens: These are common additives used to stop the formation of mold in foods. The addition of parabens trick you into thinking your food is fresher than it is. They have been linked to hormonal imbalance and breast cancer.

Potassium bromate: This is a compound that is added to breads and similar food substances to help increase the size of the food. It has been linked to cancer.

Propylene glycol: This is a thickening agent used in dairy products as well as antifreeze. Although it has been FDA-approved, if there is too much of it in the body, it can become dangerous. Some of the side effects related to ingestion of propylene glycol include depression, seizures and allergic contact dermatitis.

Propyl gallate: This is an artificial food additive which stops food from spoiling. It has been said that too much propyl gallate can cause stomach and skin issues, breathing difficultly and an increased risk of cancer.

Refined vegetable oil: A very popular part of many people's diets, refined vegetable oil is linked to heart disease and cancer. Examples of refined vegetable oils include soybean oil, canola oil, peanut oil and corn oil.

Sodium benzoate: This is a food additive that is used as a preservative in certain foods and drinks so that they can be stored for longer periods of time. It has been linked to hyperactivity in children. Research is being done into a link to cancer.

Sodium nitrate: This is a salt that is added to cured meats and other foods to prevent them from spoiling too quickly. It has been said that too much sodium nitrate can affect oxygen circulation and increase the risk of cancer.

Sulfites: Sulfites are added to food to enhance flavor and to help preserve food for longer. While some people do not react to sulphites, a great number of people who are sulfite sensitive can have an adverse reaction. These reactions include asthma and other breathing related issues.

Trans fat: Trans fat is created by adding hydrogen to vegetable oil. It is a factory-made ingredient found in deep fried foods and baked goods. It has been said that too much trans fat can increase the risk of type 2 diabetes as well as heart disease. Foods that are high in trans fats tend to be filled with chemicals that are designed to over stimulate your dopamine emitters, giving you a profound sense of wellbeing while you are eating the food, similar in a lot of ways, to a drug. You often become addicted to such foods and ingesting them can result in significant weight gain.

Polysorbate 60: This emulsifier is often derived from petroleum and is widely used. This waxy substance cannot spoil and is used as a replacement for dairy products in baked goods and other liquid products.

Magnesium sulphate: While it is generally recognized as safe by the FDA, very high doses have been shown to be fatal in human beings, and it has been linked to cancer in laboratory animals.

Has this food been changed from its original form?

We are meant to be eating food in its original state, exactly the way it has grown from the earth. This means that any alterations to our food will render it less healthy and will result in weight gain, illness and disease. Any food that has been altered should be avoided, including bread that has been refined by having the bran and germ removed or vegetables that have been stir fried, for example. Cooking should always be kept to a minimum because the process actually drains food of all its natural nutrients.

Have any components of this food been manufactured in a lab?

Unfortunately, so much of our food now is created rather than grown. The modern food production process has changed from farming and rearing to science experiments done in a lab. This means that this lab-created food has been artificially manufactured to taste good and contains no real ingredients and nutritional value. To simplify it, if you're looking at a product that has a label with a long list of ingredients that you cannot even pronounce, then it's best not to buy that food.

Processed foods are pretty much everywhere and are probably the vast majority of the food that you currently buy and eat. So, why are foods that possess the aforementioned features so bad for you? How does the addition of these processes during the manufacturing of foods affect your body?

The thing is, processed foods aren't bad per se, and there are times where they can be healthy if there is limited processing. Pasteurization, for example, is a process that destroys pathogenic microorganisms which are potentially very harmful. So, it is a process that actually makes milk healthier for you, and hence safer to consume than non-pasteurized milk.

The trick is to avoid certain ultra-processed foods that are manufactured to turn them into taste bombs with absolutely no nutritional value. It is best to avoid foods that possess no nutritional benefits whatsoever, such as deep fried foods and potato chips. If you are eating steamed kale, a very healthy food, that has been slightly processed by cooking to make it palatable, the positives outweigh the negatives. However, if you are eating a donut, a highly processed and highly unhealthy food product, then the negatives outweigh the positives. In other words, always go for foods rather than food products.

This is why the clean eating diet is so effective. By eating clean, you start to teach your body to become less dependent on unnatural processed foods and instead you learn how to gain more energy and vitality through natural means. And through this process, your body and mind are left feeling happier and healthier.

CHAPTER 2

The Benefits of Clean Eating

Like most people, you might have tried many diets over the years and failed, swearing you'll never try again. The truth is that we're all looking for the best way to lose weight, and we're all pretty much willing to try diet after diet to find it. Eventually you get to a stage when you're sick of the diets, and you're tired of never getting it right. So what makes the clean eating diet different from any of the other diets that you've tried and failed over the years? How can you be sure that this diet is the one that will provide you with the results you desire where other diets failed to produce any real benefit?

What's the difference between this diet and the others? Research. Clean eating has been scientifically proven through stringent research to aid in the improvement of health as well as the attainment of healthy, balanced weight loss. We've put together a list of 10 reasons why clean eating is so good for you:

You'll lose weight and keep it off. One of the best things about clean eating is that it's not a diet but rather a way of living. So even though you will lose weight through the process you will also keep it off forever if you continue to eat this way.

You will have a better immune system. The more nutritious your food is, the stronger your immune system will be. This means that you will be able to fight off illness more quickly and easily.

You'll have more energy. The more processed and packaged your food is the more sluggish and lethargic you'll feel. Over the years we have accustomed our bodies to getting energy through the wrong avenues, such as by drinking caffeine-laden drinks and consuming copious amounts of sugar. However, while your energy levels will increase from the effects of these stimulants, you will also experience a crash and a drop in energy the moment they leave the body. By introducing your body to more natural foods, you will start finding that not only are you more energetic but that this energy is long-lasting and slow releasing.

You'll think more clearly. By eating unprocessed, healthy and hearty foods, you will help to keep your brain functioning at its full capacity.

You'll sleep better. The reason that so many people battle to get a good night's rest is because the natural state of their hormones has been tampered with. Constant high energy and low energy fluctuations cause an imbalance within the body which in turn makes it hard for the body to shut down when you want to go to sleep. The complete set of vitamins and minerals that you'll get from clean eating will help to regulate your hormonal system throughout the day and allow you to sleep better at night.

Your mood will improve. The better you eat, the better your sense of positivity and wellbeing will be. You'll be more energized while still retaining a sense of calm. On a personal note, I can definitely see how my own mood has gotten better since I changed to a clean eating diet. I was very easily annoyed and frustrated before, whereas now, I have a clearer sense of the world around me now. I'm able to look for solutions when a problem comes up rather than getting frustrated and walking away from the situation.

Your skin will glow. The idea is simple, you are what you eat. So if you're eating clean, then your skin will look clean. A natural glow to the skin is one of the best ways of looking young and healthy. I have a friend who had mild, but persistent acne. She followed a clean eating diet for just 10 days and was astounded to find that her acne cleared up on its own without the use of prescription medication.

Your hair will shine. Just as above, it is important to note that what you put into your body will naturally have an impact on both the inside and the outside. So if you're eating food that is natural and clean, then you will start to see it have an effect on the way you look. This includes a healthier and shinier head of hair.

You'll enjoy better workouts. The better you eat, the more energy you will have, which in turn will help you to put more effort into your exercise when you are training. The right type of food will not only help you to work out better but will also help you to build muscle, lose weight and boost your recovery time between workouts.

You'll save money. The more you spend on healthy eating, the less you'll end up spending in health care costs. You'll find yourself going to the doctor less and spending less on medication and hospital bills. You can even reduce your risk of heart disease and certain cancers by eating clean.

The difference between the calories contained in an apple and, for example, a donut is far more subtle than the difference between the numbers themselves. Depending on the size, an apple might even have the same number of calories as a donut! Why, then, is an apple, which is part of a clean eating diet, better than a donut if it has the exact same number of calories? It is because an apple contains fiber and vitamins and minerals as well as other components that are good for the health of your body. Whereas, a donut contains very little nutritional value and is little more than a huge helping of heavily processed sugars. So, eating a single apple will satisfy your hunger more than a donut because, despite the equivalent number of calories, it contains a lot more nutrients. You'll satisfy your hunger with less food and therefore lose weight quicker.

The logic behind clean eating is simple. The consumption of wholesome foods boosts your metabolism and helps you eat less, and helps you lose weight while simultaneously improving your health. This is what sets it apart from the other diets. The logic behind it is simple and effective, and you can get observable results, usually the loss of about one pound every day or perhaps every two days, within less than two weeks!

CHAPTER 3

The Ten Day Diet Plan

So now that you've got a better understanding of what clean eating is all about and what benefits this type of diet can have on your body, it's time to look at how you can start to implement it into your own life. While this is a way of life and not a traditional diet or a fad, we wanted to present you with a ten day plan to help you move into this way of eating with ease. Why? Because it's important that you ease into a new lifestyle instead of diving head first into it. It's good for you allow your body time to fully adjust to this new way of eating and to create habits that will last you a lifetime. We know that by the end of the ten days you'll want to continue with this lifestyle for good, but for now we simply ask that you dedicate ten days to making the change. You need ten days to help rid your body of toxins and to overcome the cravings that you have built up for sugar and processed foods.

Step 1: Decide on a start date.
Step 2: Clean out your kitchen and fridge of all processed foods and any foods that contain additives.
Step 3: Go shopping.
Step 4: Begin the ten day process.

Don't worry; we're going to help you with as much information as possible. Next, we'll go through all the foods that are recommended to eat in these ten days, what foods you are allowed in moderation and other tips and tricks that might be of help to you.

Foods that are highly recommended during the ten days:

Lean protein: ground turkey, chicken breasts, wild salmon, eggs, game meat, cod, pork chops, scallops.

Grains: quinoa, wild brown rice, whole wheat bread.

Fatty proteins: avocado, coconut, walnut, cashews, almonds, nut flour, all natural peanut butter, seeds, salmon, bluefish, trout, mussels.

Flours: spelt flour, wheat flour, oat flour, chickpea flour, rice flour, quinoa flour.

Fruit: melon, apple, papaya, pear, raspberry, blueberry, blackberry, cherry, mango, guava, orange, passion fruit, strawberry, tangerine, tomato, grapefruit.

Vegetables: broccoli, cauliflower, artichoke, Brussels sprouts, asparagus, carrots, onions, shallots, garlic, cucumbers, squash, zucchini, pumpkins, avocado.

Leaves: kale, collard greens, spinach, arugula, beet greens, chard, turnip greens, endive, lettuce, mustard greens, watercress, garlic chives, cabbage.

Super foods: Goji, cacao, spirulina, chia, flax.

Dairy: unsweetened almond milk, unsweetened rice milk, Greek yogurt, cottage cheese.

Nuts: walnuts, almonds, macadamia nuts, hazelnuts and pecans

Foods allowed in moderation during the ten days:

Use oils sparingly throughout the ten days. This includes sunflower oil, coconut oil, walnut oil, avocado oil, olive oil, grape seed oil and pumpkin seed oil.
Sugar free maple syrup.
Mackerel (careful, it is high in mercury).
Sweeter fruits such as bananas, dates, figs and persimmons.

Tips and tricks:

Don't forget to drink enough water every day. It is important to stay hydrated to help your body through the detoxification and elimination process. This will also play a big role in weight loss.

Listen to your body and make sure you are getting enough food every day. Remember that just because you are trying to lose weight doesn't mean you have to starve yourself. You will naturally lose weight throughout the clean eating process, and because it is a way of a life and not a diet, you will also keep this weight off.

Learn how to eat mindfully, and take the time to chew your food slowly. We spend far too much time eating in front of the computer or TV that we don't even realize what we are eating. Take the time to really think about what you are putting in your body and to say thank you for the food that you have.

Use seasoning and spices to your advantage. Use things like Himalayan sea salt, cinnamon, cayenne pepper, wasabi, black pepper, rosemary, basil, thyme, coriander, curry paste, ginger, onion flakes, parsley, sage, garlic, etc. to give your food extra flavor without the extra calories.

Don't exceed two fruits a day, because although fruit is good for you, it is still high in sugar. While the sugar in fruits is natural, it is still the case of too much of a good thing being bad for you. So limit yourself to one or two fruits a day to stay within a healthy sugar range.

Eat a few small meals throughout the day rather than three big meals. This will help to speed up your metabolism and allow your body time to fully absorb all the nutrients it needs.

Try to eat as many raw foods as you can. The cooking process can often be quite harsh on certain foods, and a lot of important nutrients and minerals get lost in the process. While you are still allowed to cook on the clean eating diet, try to include as many raw foods as possible, especially vegetables.

Try to cook your own food as much as possible. When you make your own food from scratch you get to see exactly what goes in it and how it is being made. When you do eat out, try to be as mindful as possible about what you are eating and stick to foods that fall under 'clean eating'.

Keep things simple. One of the many reasons why people fail when trying to lose weight is that they try to complicate things too much. There are so many things you can eat while on the clean eating diet. All you have to do is eat foods that are unprocessed and that have no additives included. That's it. There's no special formula and no hidden secrets. Don't get overwhelmed by the process and just keep it simple.

When you go shopping, look at labels. The longer the list of ingredients the more likely that food is going to be unhealthy for you. Food ingredients should be short and recognizable. If you don't know what half the words mean it is because it's been made in a factory and all those words stand for a chemical. Keep it simple and always ask yourself: 'Where did this food come from? Are the ingredients natural or processed?"

CHAPTER 4

Tasty Clean Eating Recipes

A lot of people are put off by the clean eating diet because they assume that following this diet means eating bland food. However, this is far from the truth. Clean eating isn't just a diet; it's a veritable way of life. Just to show you how much variety you get while eating clean and just how many delicious dishes you can make, we've put together some delicious ideas for clean eating recipes. You are welcome to play around with these as much as you want. You can take out ingredients that you don't like and add in ones you do like, as long as they are part of the clean eating food list. Remember to make the process fun and to never stop enjoying what you eat. It's all about finding what works well for your body and learning how to enjoy food in a healthier way. Don't be afraid to experiment in the kitchen.

Quinoa Salad With Asparagus, Dates And Orange

This is a tasty and easy to put together dish that combines whole grains and tangy fruit. Not only is this dish delicious, it is an excellent source of fiber and protein! Quinoa is packed with a large number of vitamins and minerals including magnesium, iron, potassium, calcium and copper. It's a great base for many dishes.

Salad ingredients:

2 cups of water

½ a teaspoon of salt

½ a cup of finely chopped onion (white)

1 teaspoon of olive oil

1 cup of uncooked quinoa

1 large, sectioned orange

¼ cup of chopped pecans

2 tablespoons of minced onion (red)

5 pitted and chopped dates

½ lb 2 inch long steamed and chilled asparagus slices

½ a diced jalapeno pepper

Dressing ingredients:

1 tablespoon of extra virgin olive oil

2 tablespoons fresh lemon juice

¼ quarter teaspoon of salt

¼ teaspoon of fresh ground black pepper

2 tablespoons of chopped mint (fresh)

1 minced garlic clove

Mint sprigs for garnishing

Method:

Salad

1. Heat the olive oil in a non-stick pan over medium-high heat.
2. Add the white onions and sauté for two minutes, followed by the quinoa which you will sauté for five more minutes.
3. Add the water and the salt and bring the mixture to a boil, then cover the pan and reduce the heat.
4. Let this simmer for about 15 minutes, and then remove from heat and let it stand until all of the water has been absorbed.
5. Place the mixture into a large bowl, add the rest of the ingredients and gently toss.

Dressing

1. Combine the lemon juice, olive oil, salt, pepper and garlic in a small bowl. Stir with a whisk.
2. Add the dressing to the salad and toss gently.
3. Sprinkle the fresh chopped mint and garnish with the mint sprigs.

Fresh Vegetables With Romesco Sauce And Poached Eggs

This dish is an excellent combination of taste and nutrition. Romesco is a nut and red pepper based sauce that originates from Tarragon in Northeastern Spain. It's very popular because not only is it very tasty and easy to implement into many dishes but it's also incredibly easy to make. It is possibly one of the best brunch ideas you will find.

Brussels sprouts are an excellent source of vitamins and nutrients, including vitamin C and vitamin K. They are a very good source of several other nutrients including folate, manganese, vitamin B6, dietary fiber, choline, vitamin B1, potassium, and omega-3 fatty acids.

Romesco Sauce ingredients:

1 cup of roasted, crushed tomatoes

1 cup of drained, roasted red peppers

1 crushed garlic clove

½ cup of slivered almonds (raw)

Himalayan sea salt to taste

2 teaspoons of paprika

1 teaspoon of cayenne pepper (if you want the sauce hot!)

Other ingredients:

6 fresh eggs

2 oz of asparagus

3 carrots

3 ½ oz of Brussels sprouts

3 sweet potatoes

1 onion

3 ½ oz of uncooked spinach

1 teaspoon of extra virgin olive oil

Method:

1. Preheat your oven to 400 F.
2. Rinse all of the vegetables clean, and chop them up.
3. Spread the vegetables on a baking sheet and coat them in oil and salt.
4. Roast until they are tender (this should take about forty minutes).
5. During the roasting process, combine the ingredients for the sauce in a blender or food processor and pulse until they have combined to form a thick sauce, and then pour this sauce into a bowl and store in the fridge.
6. Poach the eggs: Fill a pot with about two cups of water and a tablespoon of vinegar and break the eggs open into a ramekin. Once the water has come to a boil, stir it gently in a consistent motion. Pour the eggs into the water slowly, keep them together with the spoon. Cook until the egg white is opaque.
7. Now simply combine all of the ingredients and plate them.

Fennel And Spinach Salad With Shrimp And Balsamic Vinaigrette

Spinach is by far one of the best vegetables you can include in your diet. It is high in iron and has a mild taste that allows it to be the ideal base for any kind of salad. Spinach has an extremely high nutritional value and is rich in antioxidants. It is a good source of vitamins A, B2, C and K, and also contains magnesium, manganese, folate, iron, calcium and potassium.

Fennel is a great source of vitamin C, fiber and folate. Vitamin C helps to neutralize free radicals in the body and boost the overall health of the immune system. The fiber content in fennel works to lower high cholesterol and improve heart health. Folate, a B vitamin, can help reduce the risk of heart attack and stroke.

Ingredients:

1 lb pound peeled and deveined jumbo shrimp

2 cups of thinly sliced fennel bulb

1 cup of halved, firm grape tomatoes

½ cup of thinly sliced onion (red)

1 (9 oz) package of fresh baby spinach

2 tablespoons of shallots, finely chopped

3 tablespoons of extra virgin olive oil

1 tablespoon of balsamic vinegar

1 teaspoon of Dijon mustard

¼ teaspoon of fresh ground black pepper

¼ teaspoon of salt

Method:

1. Sauté the shrimp in olive oil for two minutes, turning them over once after one minute.
2. Mix the fennel, grape tomatoes, onion and baby spinach into a bowl.
3. Combine the rest of the ingredients, except for the shrimp, in another bowl and gently stir with a whisk.
4. Mix all of the ingredients together and toss well.

Oatmeal Power Bowl

The Oatmeal Power Bowl is one of the healthiest and not to mention tastiest breakfasts you can eat. Full of vitamins and fiber to give your metabolism that all important kick start in the morning, the Oatmeal Power Bowl is the perfect mix of taste and texture. One of the best ingredients in this bowl is the chia seeds, which are tiny black seeds from a South American plant called Salvia Hispanica.

These seeds may be small, but they contain some powerful properties that give you energy and provide you with antioxidants and added fiber. Chia has twice the amount of protein than most other grains and has five times more calcium than milk. In addition, it has of high levels of omega-3 and omega-6 fatty acids and potassium. This has become my own favorite breakfast and one that my whole family has come to love.

Ingredients:

1 mashed ripe banana (the riper the better!)

2 tablespoons of chia seeds

1/3 of a cup of rolled oats

¼ teaspoon of cinnamon

2/3 of a cup of almond milk

¼ cup of water

1 tablespoon of ground flax

Garnish ingredients:

Almonds (soaked)

Pepita seeds

Hemp hearts

Cinnamon

Toasted coconut

Nut butter

Ginger

Allspice

Method:

1. Before going to sleep at night, mash the bananas in a bowl until they acquire a smooth texture.
2. Stir all the other ingredients, from the chia seeds to the water, into the mixture, cover and refrigerate overnight.
3. In the morning, heat the mixture in a pot on medium-high heat until it begins to simmer.
4. Reduce heat to medium low and stir frequently until it acquires an even thickness and is hot throughout.
5. Add the flax.
6. Pour into a bowl, and add the garnishes to taste!

Chicken With Brussels Sprouts And Mustard Sauce

Chicken is the all-purpose meat, much like spinach is the all-purpose vegetable. This dish is a zesty and healthy choice for dinner or even lunch if you are looking for something substantial during the day! Brussels sprouts include a huge amount of vitamin C and vitamin K and contain many healthy nutrients for the body. Combining Brussels sprouts with chicken means that you are creating a meal that has all the protein, nutrients and vitamins your body needs.

Ingredients:

2 tablespoons of olive oil

4 (6 oz) halves of skinned and boneless chicken breast

½ a teaspoon of salt

¼ teaspoon of black pepper (freshly ground)

¾ cup of chicken broth (fat free and low sodium, remember that you are on a diet!)

¼ cup of apple cider (unfiltered)

2 tablespoons of Dijon mustard (whole grain)

2 tablespoons of olive butter

1 tablespoon of flat leaf parsley (chopped)

12 oz trimmed and halved Brussels sprouts

Method:

1. Preheat the oven to about 450 F.
2. Put an oven proof pan on high heat and add half of the oil.
3. Sprinkle the chicken with salt and pepper and place it on the pan.
4. Cook for about three minutes, then turn over and place into the oven.
5. Bake for around nine minutes.
6. Remove chicken from the pan, place pan on medium high heat and add half cup each of chicken broth and cider.
7. Reduce heat to medium-low and let simmer for about four minutes.
8. Add mustard, one tablespoon of olive butter and parsley, and whisk the ingredients in a bowl.
9. Heat the rest of the butter and oil in a large nonstick pan over medium-high heat.
10. Sauté Brussels sprouts in oil and butter for two minutes.
11. Add remaining broth and salt, cover and let cook for about four minutes.
12. Plate Brussels sprouts with chicken and serve.

Vanilla Almond Chia Breakfast Pudding

There are very few foods that one can actually call super foods. Chia is one of them. Discovered by the ancient Mayans and Aztecs, this super food is an excellent source of anti-oxidants as well as omega 3, calcium and fiber, making it an excellent food to start your day off with! Just add this dish to your growing list of clean eating breakfast foods. Remember when we told you that you'd hardly notice that you were on a diet while eating clean? Dishes like this are the reason why.

Ingredients:

2 cups of unsweetened almond milk
½ a cup of chia seeds
½ a teaspoon of vanilla extract
2 tablespoons of maple syrup or honey
(go for pure maple syrup or raw honey)

For the toppings, add any fruits that are in season and nuts high in essential fatty acids and vitamin E such as walnuts, almonds, hazelnuts or pecans

Method:

1. Combine the almond milk, chia seeds, vanilla extract and maple syrup or honey.
2. Mix until the mixture acquires a thick consistency.
3. Cover the mixture and store it in the fridge overnight (or for at least an hour).
4. Stir well before serving, and remember to add all of the toppings!

Arugula, Grape And Sunflower Seed Salad

Salads are perhaps the staple meal of anyone that is looking to lose some major weight. The same is true for those following a clean eating diet. Salads are low in calories but pack a huge nutritional punch, providing you with all of the essential vitamins and minerals you need, allowing you to give your body its fill of daily nutrients without overloading on unnecessary calories. The arugula, grape and sunflower seed salad is a great choice if you are looking for a light lunch that can be both made and eaten without much of a fuss. It doesn't hurt that it tastes great too, and is one of the simplest and healthiest salads.

Ingredients:

3 tablespoons of vinegar (red wine)
1 teaspoon of honey
1 teaspoon of pure maple syrup
½ teaspoon of stone grounded mustard
2 teaspoons of grape seed oil
7 cups of baby arugula (loosely packed)

2 cups of halved red grapes
2 tablespoons of sunflower seed kernels (toasted)
1 teaspoon of chopped, fresh thyme
2 pinches each of salt and fresh ground black pepper

Method:

1. Combine the vinegar, honey, maple syrup and mustard in a bowl.
2. Add oil gradually, mixing it in with a whisk.
3. Add the arugula, thyme and all the other ingredients in a separate bowl.
4. Sprinkle the vinegar mixture over the arugula.
5. Sprinkle salt and pepper.
6. Toss well.

Apple Mug Muffin

A sweet dish that fits in perfectly with all food you consume while following the ten day plan. Who said you can't spoil yourself while dieting? The Apple Mug Muffin is comfort food, plain and simple. Apples are known for being high in fiber, and the soluble fiber found in apples binds with fats in the intestine, which translates into lower cholesterol levels and a healthier you. Studies have also shown that women who eat at least one apple a day are less likely to develop type 2 diabetes.

Ingredients:

1 tablespoon of butter (grass fed only) or coconut oil
2 tablespoons of applesauce (unsweetened)
1 egg
¼ teaspoon of vanilla extract
4 tablespoons of maple syrup
3 tablespoons of almond flour
½ a teaspoon of cinnamon
A pinch of baking powder
A pinch of salt

Ingredients for the Streusel topping:

1 tablespoon of finely chopped apple
A pinch of crumbled walnuts
A pinch of cold butter

Method:

1. Preheat the oven to about 350 F.
2. Grease the mug you will cook the muffin in with the butter.
3. Whisk the applesauce, egg, vanilla and maple syrup into the mug until they have formed a thick mixture.

4. Add the almond flour, cinnamon and baking powder as well as the salt and stir the mixture for about one minute.
5. Add the topping after mixing it with your fingers.
6. Place the mug into the oven for about twenty five minutes.

Vegetable Hash With Poached Egg

A lot of people say that there is no substitute for high calorie foods like pizza and that people who enjoy these foods will have to simply suffer in silence if they want to lose a significant amount of weight in a short period of time. This is simply not true. Vegetable hash is a wholesome and hearty dish that can serve as a great substitute for pizza as well as pasta.

Zucchini is a good source of protein, vitamin A, vitamin C and vitamin K. It is also an excellent source of dietary fiber, riboflavin and vitamin B6. Yellow squash is high in vitamin C, iron, folate and beta carotene. Beta carotene is an antioxidant that helps protect your body against damage from pollutants and free radicals.

Ingredients:

2 tablespoons of olive oil
1 cup of chopped onion (preferably a sweet onion like Vidalia)
1 cup of quarter inch slices of small red potato
1 teaspoon of herbes de Provence (dried)
1 cup of zucchini (diced)
1 cup of yellow squash (diced)
1 cup of half inch pieces of trimmed green beans

2 cups of chopped tomatoes with the seeds removed
2 cups of chives (thinly sliced)
2 tablespoons of flat leaf parsley (chopped)
1 tablespoon of white vinegar
4 eggs (large)
1 ounce of shredded parmesan cheese

Method:

1. Heat a large pan over medium-high heat. Coat the pan in oil.
2. Add the herbes de Provence along with the onions and potatoes.
3. Spread the mixture until it is evenly spread in the pan, and let it cook without stirring for about four minutes.
4. Reduce the flame until it is at medium and add the zucchini, squash, beans, salt and about half of the black pepper by stirring it in.
5. Let it cook for about three minutes.

6. Remove the pan from the heat, and let it stand for five minutes.
7. Stir in the parsley as well as the chives and tomatoes.
8. Add water to a separate large pan until it is about two thirds full.
9. Bring the water to a boil.
10. Reduce the heat and let the water simmer.
11. Add the vinegar.
12. Break the eggs into custard cups.
13. Pour the eggs into the pan.
14. Cook for three minutes.
15. Remove the eggs carefully using a slotted spoon.
16. Divide the squash mixture into four even portions.
17. Add one egg on top of each portion.
18. Sprinkle egg with remaining pepper and add parmesan cheese.

Tofu Quiche

What's this? A great breakfast recipe without eggs? Impossible? Not at all. This is a breakfast dish without eggs that tastes amazing and is incredibly healthy for you. The tofu quiche is further proof of the versatility and diversity of the clean eating diet. Tofu, which is derived from soybean curds, is naturally low in calories, cholesterol-free and is a great source of protein, iron and calcium. Soy, the primary component of tofu, is a complete source of dietary protein, providing all of the essential amino acids needed for a healthy diet.

Ingredients for the crust:

3 cups of grated potato
2 tablespoons of grass-fed butter
(substitute vegan butter or olive oil if
you want to avoid animal products)

A pinch each of salt and pepper

Ingredients for the filling of the quiche:

12 oz of silken tofu, extra firm, which
has been patted dry
2 tablespoons of yeast
3 tablespoons of hummus
3 chopped cloves of garlic

2 thinly sliced leeks OR one diced onion
¾ of a cup of halved cherry tomatoes
1 cup of broccoli (chopped)
Salt and pepper to taste

Method:

1. Preheat the oven to about 450 F.
2. Add the grated potatoes to a pie dish.
3. Drizzle with melted butter and a pinch each of salt and pepper.
4. Toss the contents of the pie pan and then even them out with your fingers.
5. Bake for approximately twenty-five minutes.
6. While the potatoes are baking, add the vegetables to a baking sheet.
7. Add the olive oil and salt and pepper and toss.
8. Add to the oven with the crust.
9. Once you remove the crust, lower the heat to 400 F.
10. Bake the vegetables for another twenty minutes.
11. Add tofu to a blender with hummus, yeast and salt and black pepper to taste while veggies are baking.
12. Once veggies are baked, remove them and lower oven temp to 375 F.
13. Mix veggies with tofu mixture.
14. Toss, add to crust and even out.
15. Bake for around 30 minutes.
16. Serve and enjoy!

Lemony Chicken Kebabs

Add some Middle Eastern flavor to your diet! Chicken is a lean protein that can trigger protein synthesis in the body and aid in the building of muscle tissue.

Depending on the availability of amino acids, the body is always in a state of muscle loss and gain. When you replenish that pool of building blocks by eating protein, you are able to promote muscle development.

The data shows us that those who eat more protein have more lean muscle mass. High-protein diets are also known to boost fat loss because protein reduces hunger. Protein is very filling, and when you eat more of it, you are more quickly satisfied and eat fewer calories.

Ingredients:

3 tablespoons of fresh squeezed lemon juice

1 tablespoon of minced garlic

1 ½ tablespoons of dried oregano

¾ of a tablespoon of salt

¾ of a tablespoon of black pepper (fresh ground)

3 tablespoons of extra virgin olive oil

24 oz of chicken breast cut into one and a half inch cubes

2 cups of fresh parsley leaves

1 cup of chopped cherry tomatoes

Method:

1. Mix two tablespoons of lemon juice, 1 tablespoon of garlic, a teaspoon of oregano, a pinch of salt and a pinch of black pepper in a bowl.
2. Stir one tablespoon of oil in with a whisk.
3. Add the chicken and stir.
4. Cover and leave in fridge for two hours to marinate.
5. Remove the chicken and thread onto four skewers ten inches long.
6. Cook for six minutes in a grill pan on high heat turning frequently.
7. Mix the remaining juice, oregano, garlic, salt and pepper in another bowl.
8. Mix the remaining oil in with a whisk.
9. Add parsley and tomatoes, then toss.
10. Plate chicken on top of salad and serve.

Shakshuka

This Israeli dish is an interesting and flavorful combination of eggs and tomato sauce. It is dish that it is healthy and delicious and can be eaten for breakfast or dinner. Tomatoes are an excellent source of vitamins A and C, as well as folic acid. They contain a wide array of beneficial nutrients and antioxidants, including alpha-lipoic acid, lycopene, choline, folic acid, beta-carotene and lutein.

Alpha-lipoic acid helps the body to convert glucose into energy. Some evidence suggests that alpha-lipoic acid can help in blood glucose control and may even help preserve brain and nerve tissue. Lycopene is the antioxidant that gives tomatoes their rich red color. Lycopene has been shown to lower the risk of prostate cancer. Choline helps with sleep, muscle movement, learning and memory.

Ingredients:

1 tablespoon of olive oil
½ an onion (peeled and diced)
1 minced clove of garlic
1 medium sized bell pepper (chopped)
4 cups of diced tomato
2 tablespoons of tomato paste

1 teaspoon each of chili powder, cumin and paprika
A pinch of cayenne pepper
A pinch of sugar
6 eggs
1/2 a tablespoon of chopped parsley as a garnish

Method:

1. Heat a large pan.
2. Warm the olive oil in the pan.
3. Sauté the onions until they soften.
4. Add garlic, and then continue to sauté till the mixture becomes aromatic.
5. Add bell pepper and sauté for another six minutes.
6. Add tomatoes and tomato paste, and stir until mixture has a smooth consistency.
7. Add the seasonings according to your taste.
8. Crack the eggs open, place them evenly across the top of the mixture one at a time.
9. Cover the pan, let simmer for around twelve minutes making sure that the sauce doesn't dry out.
10. Garnish with parsley, serve with pita bread or a green salad and enjoy.

Oven Fried Sweet Potatoes

Filled to the brim with vitamins, minerals and fiber, oven fried sweet potatoes are so yummy, you just might end up serving this as the main course for dinner. Sweet potatoes are high in vitamins B6, C and D. Vitamin B6 can help to reduce the homocysteine in the body, reducing the risk of heart attacks and degenerative diseases. Vitamin C helps with wound healing and boosts collagen, which is so important for healthy skin. Vitamin D plays a very important role in the immune system and boosts overall health, especially in the winter months.

Sweet potatoes also contain iron, which helps build up your resistance to stress and ensures you have an adequate store of energy. They are an excellent source of magnesium, the relaxation and anti-stress mineral. The natural sugars in sweet potatoes are released into the bloodstream slowly without resulting in the spike in blood sugar that artificial sweeteners cause. These sugar highs can lead to fatigue and weight gain. So the next time you're in the mood for a sweet snack, think about making this dish.

Ingredients:

4 medium sized sweet potatoes cut into quarter inch slices
1 tablespoon of olive oil
A pinch each of salt and pepper
Vegetable cooking spray

1 tablespoon of fresh parsley, finely chopped
1 teaspoon of grated orange rind
1 small, minced garlic clove

Method:

1. Preheat the oven to 400 F.
2. Mix the sweet potatoes with the olive oil, salt and pepper.
3. Toss the mixture gently.
4. Coat a baking sheet with cooking spray.
5. Place the sweet potato slices in a single layer upon the baking sheet.
6. Bake the sweet potato slices for about 30 minutes (turn the slices over after fifteen minutes.
7. Mix the parsley, orange rind and garlic.
8. Stir the mixture together gently but thoroughly.
9. Sprinkle this mixture over the sweet potato slices.
10. Serve and enjoy.

CHAPTER 5

Exercise as a Supplement to Clean Eating

Clean eating is, in fact, a comprehensive and versatile lifestyle choice that provides amazing results in and of itself. But, if you want to speed up your weight loss, then it's important to supplement it with exercise.

We've put together three basic areas for you to target through a series of light to moderate exercises. All of these exercises are body weight exercises that don't require any equipment, in keeping with the back to basics nature of eating clean. Most people fall back on excuses when it comes to exercising and will tell you that they cannot exercise because they don't have enough money for a gym membership or the right equipment. Simply put, you don't need all that. All you need is the will and determination to succeed.

Upper Body

Push-ups: The push up is possibly one of the most effective and simple exercises you can do to build upper body strength. They can be performed at home, at the park or even on the basketball court, without need of much space or any specialized equipment. This exercise works your chest, shoulders and triceps. The one complaint we always get when it comes to push-ups is that after a while they might get boring or monotonous, and the most important thing when it comes to exercise is to keep it fun and different. So while push-ups in their original state are good for you there are also many variations you can try to keep the exercise varied:

The Wide Grip Push-Up: Here you start from your normal push-up position but you spread your hands wider than normal, around shoulder length. This means that your chest will get a much better workout than from a normal push-up.

The Narrow Grip Push-Up: Similar to the above, except now you bring your hands only a few inches apart from each other underneath your chest.

The Single Leg Push-Up: This is a high intensity work out that will work both the upper body and the core. Here you do your push-ups as normal only you lift one leg off the ground per set and switch legs on the next set.

The Single Arm Push-Up: This is a great way to target the direct muscles of the arms and shoulders. This is a normal push-up but using one arm at a time while placing the other arm behind your back. Don't be frustrated if you can't do this one straight away because this does require a lot of upper body strength which you might not have just yet. Keep working at it and watch as you get fitter over time.

The Clap Push-Up: This targets the chest and will also elevate the heart rate, so there is a cardiovascular element to it. Here you do your push-ups as usual but when you reach the peak of it you quickly lift your hands in midair and clap. This hard but very effective addition to the normal push-up will help you to see results quickly.

Pull-ups: Pull-ups are another excellent exercise that you can use to work the muscles in your upper body that the push up fails to target, muscles such as your biceps, rear shoulders and your upper back. This exercise can be performed by grasping a solid metal bar and pulling yourself up using only your upper body. Keep your palms facing you if you are inexperienced with this exercise, and remember to keep your body as straight as possible as you go up and down otherwise you could seriously injure yourself. Work your way up until you can do about twenty five pull-ups.

Bicep curl: Contrary to popular belief, you do not need to have dumbbells to do bicep curls. If you do not have any dumbbells at home, then simply fill up a water bottle to the weight you want and use it instead. Start off by holding the dumbbells or bottles in your hand and place your elbows against your hip bones. One side at a time, slowly lift the weight up until your forearm touches your chest.

Core

Sit ups: This is a great core exercise to include in your daily routine, one that can be done anywhere at any time. Note that this exercise is different from the crunch because it is more intense and provides you with a better all-round abdominal workout. This exercise targets your entire abdominal area with an emphasis placed on your upper abs. This exercise is performed by lying on your back with your heel placed against your buttocks and raising your upper body up until your chest touches your knees, using only the strength of your abdominal area. Start as low as you want, even with just twenty sit ups a day. Just keep your form correct, otherwise you may injure yourself. Constantly try to increase the amount that you do each day and watch as your fitness level starts to rise.

Leg raises: This exercise is another excellent way of toning up your belly area. It exercises your entire abdominal area whilst placing an emphasis on your lower abs. Since this exercise uses more body weight than a sit up, you should do about half the number of leg raises as you do sit ups. To do this exercise, sit down on the floor and place both legs out in front of you. Make sure your back is straight at all times and if it gets too much for your back, then you can also do this one lying down. Then slowly left your right leg up, hold for a few seconds and lower it down. Do the same on the other side and continue to repeat the sequence.

Plank: This is my personal favorite exercise and certainly one that you will both love and hate at the same time. Hate because it's certainly not easy, but love because it is the one that will give you the quickest results. Start by lying down in a press up position, and then push yourself up until your body forms a straight line from the shoulders to the ankles. Try holding this for at least 30 seconds your first time. Do this every single day and constantly try to hold for longer. If your body starts to shake it means it is working, so don't give up too soon. You'll be surprised at how much more you are capable of doing. Remember to constantly engage your core by sticking in your stomach.

Legs and Butt

Squats: The squat is one of the best workouts you can do for your body and since it primarily targets the thighs and the glutes. Do this right, and you will be left looking toned in your bikini or swim trunks. Let's go through a few squat variations:

The Traditional Squat: Place your legs around shoulder length apart and bend the knees slightly. Make sure your feet are pointed slightly outward rather than straight ahead. With your arms extended ahead slowly start to bend until your knees are at a ninety degree angle. Then slowly start to come up until your back is straight again. Repeat this movement. The best way to imagine this exercise is to pretend you are about to sit on an imaginary chair. Remember to do this one slowly and deliberately.

The Weight Squat: This is the same as the traditional squat except you hold a dumbbell or a water bottle to your chest as you move down.

The Single Leg Squat: This is the same as the traditional except you lift one leg at a time while going down into your squat. This is a wonderful way to work on your balance while also improving your core muscles.

Toe raises: This exercise is a good supplement to squats because it specifically targets the muscle groups that squats do not focus on, such as your calves, ankles and glutes. The exercise is really simple. All you have to do is stand with your legs shoulder length apart and raise your body up on your toes and descend back down again. Work your way up to fifty of these a day.

Cardio

An additional area of exercise that you may want to focus on is cardiovascular exercise. This is essentially exercise that improves your lung capacity and the strength of your heart. A great way to improve cardiovascular health is to go jogging. Try to complete one mile every two days, even if you are not able to run all the way. If you feel tired during your run, simply slow down to a walk until you recover your stamina. Walking and running is a great way to lose weight and keep your heart healthy. If you stick to it, you will see a great improvement over time. Best of all, it's completely free.

Some other great cardiovascular activities that don't cost money are walking the dog, gardening, skipping, dancing and even shopping at a large mall where you have to do a great deal of walking.

Conclusion

Thank you again for downloading this book!

Clean eating is a way of life. It is not a fad or a quick-fix diet. Through healthy choices and good habits, you can completely transform the way you look and feel. It's all about going back to the basics and eating food that is fresh, organic and whole. All we are asking is that you give it ten days. Ten days where you stick by it completely. Ten days is enough time for your body to rid itself of all the toxins and impurities that have built up over the years. The first few days might be hard, and you may start off feeling worse as your body tries to rid itself from these contaminations. However once the ten days are up, you'll feel like a whole new person, and I guarantee you that you'll want to eat clean for the rest of your life.

Good luck on this exciting new journey!

Finally, if you enjoyed this book, then I'd like to ask you for a favor, would you be kind enough to leave a review for this book on Amazon? It'd be greatly appreciated!

Be sure to check out our website at www.thetotalevolution.com for more information.

Thank you!

Our Other Books

Below you'll find some of our other books that are popular on Amazon.com and the international sites.

Master Cleanse: How To Do A Natural Detox The Right Way And Lose Weight Fast

Mayo Clinic Diet: A Proven Diet Plan For Lifelong Weight Loss

Glycemic Index Diet: A Proven Diet Plan For Weight Loss and Healthy Eating With No Calorie Counting

Dukan Diet: A High Protein Diet Plan To Help You Lose Weight And Keep It Off For Life

Wheat Belly: The Anti-Diet - A Guide To Gluten Free Eating And A Slimmer Belly

IIFYM: Flexible Dieting - Sculpt The Perfect Body While Eating The Foods You Love

Mediterranean Diet: 101 Ultimate Mediterranean Diet Recipes To Fast Track Your Weight Loss & Help Prevent Disease

Acid Reflux Diet: A Beginner's Guide To Natural Cures And Recipes For Acid Reflux, GERD And Heartburn

Hypothyroidism Diet: Natural Remedies & Foods To Boost Your Energy & Jump Start Your Weight Loss

It Starts With Food: A 30 Day Diet Plan To Reset Your Body, Lose Weight And Become A Healthier You